MEN EXERCISES FOR A GOOD SEXUAL HEALTH:

Exercises to help boost men sex life

Matthew Woods

TABLE OF CONTENTS

INTRODUCTION

You know that working out is good for your health. But did you know that hitting the gym could also help you have better sex? "Working out three to four times a week can do a lot to help your sexual technique, flexibility, and endurance," says Pete McCall, MS, an exercise physiologist and personal trainer for the American Council on Exercise (ACE).

Engaging in regular physical activity can have a positive impact on men's sexual health by improving blood circulation, boosting testosterone levels, enhancing endurance, and promoting overall well-being. While there is no specific "best" exercise for improving sex, a combination of cardiovascular workouts, strength training, and pelvic floor exercises can contribute to better sexual performance and satisfaction. Here are some exercises that men can incorporate into their fitness routine to support their sexual health:

CARDIOVASCULAR EXERCISES

Your heart beats faster. You breathe more rapidly and deeply. And you sweat. Well, that's probably because you've been moving the large muscles in your legs, arms and hips over a sustained period of time. When these major muscles are involved in exercise, there is increased rate of respiration to produce energy. In turn, the need for more oxygen leads to increased breathing and heart rate. And such a form of activity is called cardiovascular exercise or cardio in short. Cardiovascular exercises increase blood flow, which is crucial for maintaining healthy erectile function and sexual arousal.

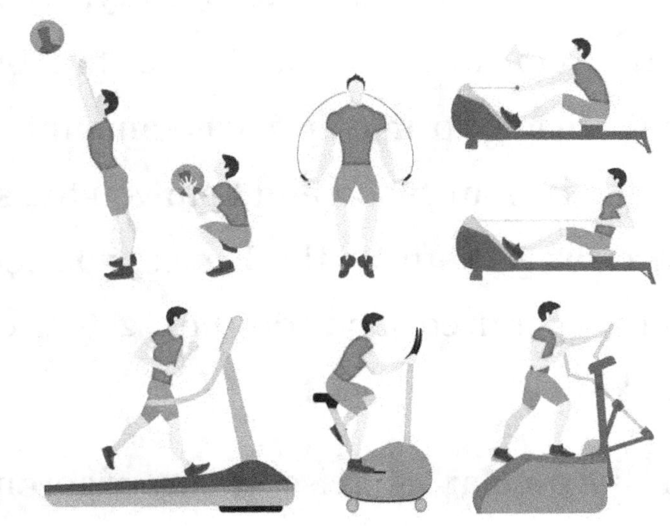

What is cardiovascular exercise?

Also called aerobic or endurance exercise, cardiovascular exercise is any form of activity that uses aerobic metabolism. That is, during the activity, oxygen is heavily involved in the cellular reactions that produce the energy necessary to sustain the activity. Your heart rate increases and you breathe more deeply to maximize the amount of oxygen in your blood and help you to use more oxygen efficiently. Hence, you feel more energized and do not get tired quickly.

Cardiovascular exercise is any vigorous activity that increases heart rate and respiration and raises oxygen and blood flow throughout the body while using large muscle groups of the body repetitively and rhythmically. Such activity progressively challenges your most vital internal body organs and improves the function and performance of the heart, lungs and circulatory system. Cardio improves many aspects of health, including heart health, mental health, mood, sleep, weight regulation and metabolism.

Actually, the heart becomes more efficient with every beat as it pumps oxygen-carrying blood, the lungs more effective in taking in oxygen, and the muscles more equipped to use more oxygen. Still, as the breathing and heart rate increase, the surge should not be so much as to make you feel that you need to stop and rest. In the course of cardio such as speed walking, cycling, swimming, running or speed climbing, if you experience a strong urge to stop and rest, unusual pain or alarming symptoms, then you have to stop immediately and seek medical attention.

But for an exercise to be considered cardio, it must raise your heart rate and breathing rate into the moderate to vigorous intensity level (at least 50-percent of the normal rate) for a minimum of 10 minutes. That is why activities undertaken to improve strength, such as resistance exercise, using weight machines, lifting weights, and core workouts are NOT considered as cardio because they do not raise the heart rate throughout the period of exercise.

Exercises or activities such as Brisk walking, Running, jogging or jogging in place, burpees, bear crawls, swimming, water aerobics, cycling/bicycling, dancing, cross-country skiing, race-walking volleyball, basketball, soccer or racquetball, rowing, kayaking, paddling or canoeing, circuit training, jumping rope, stair climbing, in-line skating, martial arts, golfing, hiking, hiit (high intensity interval training), mountain climbing, jumping jacks, squat jumps, split jumps, roller, kickboxing are all beneficial in improving cardiovascular health and sexual performance.

HIGH-INTENSITY INTERVAL TRAINING

This type of training can help improve cardiovascular fitness and boost testosterone levels, which may positively impact libido and sexual function, which is also known as HIIT.

It is a form of cardiovascular exercise that alternates between short bursts of intense exercise and periods of active rest or low-intensity exercise. HIIT workouts typically involve exercises that raise the heart rate and increase oxygen consumption, such as sprinting, jumping jacks, burpees, or cycling. The high-intensity periods usually last from

20 to 60 seconds, followed by a brief recovery period that can last from 10 seconds to 1 minute. The idea behind HIIT is to push the body to its maximum capacity for short periods of time, causing it to burn more calories and improve cardiovascular fitness. The intense periods of exercise also cause the body to continue burning calories even after the workout is finished, known as the afterburn effect or excess post-exercise oxygen consumption (EPOC). HIIT workouts can be adapted to different fitness levels and can be performed with or without equipment. They are often preferred by people who want to get the most out of their workout

in a short amount of time, as a typical HIIT session can last from 10 to 30 minutes.

High-Intensity Interval Training (HIIT) can have several effects on your sexual life including:

i.   Improved cardiovascular health: HIIT can improve heart health and blood circulation, leading to better stamina and endurance during sexual activity.

ii.   Increased energy levels: HIIT can increase energy levels, which can lead to improved sexual stamina.

iii.   Reduced fatigue: HIIT can help reduce fatigue, which can help you maintain sexual activity for longer periods of time.

iv. Increased testosterone levels: HIIT has been shown to increase testosterone levels in some studies, which can improve sexual desire and performance.

v. Improved body composition: HIIT can help improve body composition by burning fat and building lean muscle mass, which can improve self-confidence and sexual performance.

Overall, HIIT can improve physical fitness, increase energy levels, reduce fatigue, increase testosterone levels, and improve body composition, all of which can lead to improved sexual stamina.

However, it's important to note that HIIT is a high-intensity exercise and may not be appropriate for everyone, especially those with certain health conditions or fitness limitations. It's always a good idea to consult with a healthcare provider or fitness professional before starting a new exercise program.

KEGEL EXERCISES

Kegel exercises are not just for women; they can also benefit men by strengthening the pelvic floor muscles. A strong pelvic floor can lead to better control over erections and ejaculation, potentially improving sexual function and pleasure.

Doing Kegels is considered a good sex exercise for men because these exercises can help endurance and control by toning the pubococcygeus (PC) muscles, the ones that let you stop the flow of urine mid-stream. Named after Los Angeles physician Arnold Kegel, they strengthen the muscles in your body's pelvic floor, which can lead to better sex. "Men can use Kegels to delay ejaculation by contracting these muscles just before orgasm," says McCall. To do Kegels, start by interrupting the flow of urine when going to the bathroom to get familiar with your PC muscles. After that, you can do Kegels anytime and anyplace by squeezing the PC muscles. Hold for 10 seconds, relax, and do as many reps as you can before tiring. The key is to get in the habit of doing them every day so you start to see results.

How to Do Kegel Exercises

Part 1: Preparing to Do Kegel Exercises

1.   Find your pelvic muscles by stopping the flow of your urine mid-stream.

Before you do your Kegel exercises, it's important to find your pelvic muscles. These are the muscles that form the floor of your pelvic floor. The most common way to find them is to try to stop the flow of your urine midstream. This tightening is the basic move of a Kegel. Let those muscles go and resume the flow of urine and you'll have a better sense of where those Kegels are. Just remember to see a doctor before you begin your Kegel exercises if you have any medical problems that may prevent you from doing Kegels safely.

Note: Don't stop urinating midstream as your regular Kegel exercise routine. Doing Kegels while urinating more than twice a month can actually have the opposite effect, weakening the muscle. It may also cause damage to your bladder and kidneys.

2.   If you still have trouble finding your Kegels, place your finger in your vagina and squeeze your muscles.

You should feel the muscles tightening and your pelvic floor move up. Relax and you'll feel the pelvic floor move back again. Make sure your finger is clean before you insert it into your vagina.

- If you're sexually active, you can also ask your partner if they can feel you "hugging" their penis (if they have one) and letting go during sex.

3.   Use a hand mirror to find your Kegels.

If you're still having trouble locating or isolating your Kegels, place a hand mirror below your perineum, which is the skin-covered area between your vagina and your anus. Practice squeezing and relaxing what you think are your Kegel muscles. If you do this correctly, you should see your perineum contracting with each squeeze.

4.   Make sure you have an empty bladder before you begin your Kegels.

This is important. You don't want to do your Kegels with a full or a partially full bladder, or you may experience pain while you do your Kegels, as well as some leakage. Before you start your exercise routine, do a bladder check so you can perform those exercises as efficiently as possible.

5.   Concentrate on only tightening your pelvic floor muscles.

Your Kegel exercises should focus on these muscles only, so you should avoid flexing other muscles, such as your buttocks, thighs, or your abdomen, for best results. To help your concentration and the efficiency of your movements, make sure you breathe in and out as you perform each set of Kegels, instead of holding your breath. This will help you relax and get the most out of your pelvic floor exercises.

- One way to keep your muscles relaxed is to place one hand on your belly to make sure that your belly is relaxed.
- If your back or belly ache a bit after you complete a set of Kegel exercises, then it's an indication

that you're not doing them correctly.

6. Get into a comfortable position.

You can do these exercises either sitting in a chair or lying on the floor. Make sure your buttock and tummy muscles are relaxed. If you are lying down, then you should be flat on your back with your arms at your sides and your knees up and together. Keep your head down, too, to avoid straining your neck.

Part 2: Doing Kegel Exercises

1. Squeeze your pelvic floor muscles for five seconds.

When you're just starting off, this is a great exercise. You don't want to strain those muscles too much by squeezing them for too long. If five is even too long for you, you can begin by squeezing those muscles for just 2-3 seconds.

2.   Release your muscles for ten seconds.

Ideally, you should always give those pelvic floor muscles a ten-second break before you repeat the exercise. This gives them enough time to relax and to avoid strain. Count to ten before you begin the next repetition.

3.   Repeat the exercise ten times.

This can be considered one set of Kegels. If you started off by squeezing those muscles for five seconds, then squeeze them for five seconds, relax them for ten, and repeat this exercise ten times. This should be enough Kegels for one time and you should do the same set of ten 3-4 times a day, but no more.

4.   Build toward squeezing your pelvic floor muscles for ten seconds at a time.

You can increase the amount of seconds that you squeeze those muscles each week. There's no need to do them for any longer, or to do more than one set of them per time. Once you've reached the magic number of ten seconds, stick to it, and continue to do one set of 10 10-second squeezes 3-4 times a day.

5.   Do pull-in Kegels.

This is another variation on the Kegel. To perform a pull-in kegel, think of your pelvic floor muscles as a vacuum. Tense your buttocks and pull your legs up and in. Hold this position for 5 seconds and then release it. Do this 10 times in a row. It should take about 50 seconds to complete.

Part 3: Getting Results

1.   Perform your Kegel exercises at least 3-4 times a day.

If you really want them to stick, then you have to make them part of your daily routine. 3-4 times a day should be doable, as each Kegel session won't last very long, and you can find ways of fitting Kegels into your daily routine. You can aim to do them in the morning, afternoon, and evening so begin to do them like clockwork, instead of worrying about scheduling a time to do your Kegels.

2.   Fit Kegels into your busy routine.

The best part about doing Kegels is that you can do them without anyone knowing. You can do them while you're sitting at your desk in your office, having lunch with your friends, or just relaxing on the couch after a long day at work. Though lying down and isolating your Kegels and focusing hard is important for beginners, once you get the hang of isolating those muscles, you can do your Kegels almost anywhere at any time.

- You can even make a habit of doing them during a routine activity, such as checking your email.
- Once you've found a set of Kegel exercises that works for you, you should stick to this routine instead of doing even more Kegels, or doing them more strenuously. If you overdo it, you may suffer from straining when you have to urinate or move your bowels.
- Just remember that, while stopping urination midstream is a great way to locate your Kegels, you should not actually do your Kegels

routinely while urinating or you may suffer problems associated with incontinence.

3.   Expect results in a few months if you do Kegels regularly.

For some women, the results are dramatic; for others, Kegels prevent further urinary tract problems. Some women get frustrated because they do Kegels for a few weeks and don't feel any difference. Stick with it long enough to feel the changes in your body. According to the National Institutes of Health (NIH), you may be able to feel results as early as after 4-6 weeks.

4.   Ask for help if you don't think you're doing Kegels properly.

Your doctor can help you identify and isolate the correct muscles to perform the exercise. If you feel like you've been doing Kegels for a considerable amount of time, such as a few months, and have seen no results, then you should seek help from your doctor. Here's what your doctor can do for you:

- If necessary, your doctor can provide biofeedback training. This involves placing a monitoring device inside your vagina, and electrodes externally. The monitor can tell you how successful you were in contracting your pelvic floor muscles and how long you were able to hold the contraction.

- A doctor can also use electrical stimulation to help you identify the pelvic floor muscles. During this process, a small electrical current adheres to the pelvic floor muscles. When activated, the current automatically contracts the muscle. After some use, you'll most likely be able to reproduce the effect on your own.

5.   Continue doing your Kegels if you want to keep incontinence at bay.

If you want to keep those muscles strong and to keep incontinence away, then you have to continue doing your Kegels. If you stop them, even after months of exercise, your incontinence problems will return. You'll have to work to keep those muscles in shape and should be ready for the commitment.

Tips:

- In addition to strengthening your pelvic floor, Kegel exercises also help to strengthen your bowel muscles as well.

- As you become more confident with these exercises, you will find that you will be able to do them standing up. The important thing is to keep practicing throughout the day and you can do them while you're washing the dishes, waiting in a queue, or even sitting at your desk in the office, during television show commercials, or when you are stopped at a stoplight while driving.

- People assigned male at birth can also strengthen their pelvic floor muscles by doing PC muscle exercises.

- For a bit of a change from standard kegels, to stretch and relax your pelvic floor, try reverse kegel exercises.

- Try not to hold your breath, squeeze your buttocks or thighs, pull your tummy in tightly, or push down instead of squeezing and lifting.

- Pregnant people can perform kegel exercises.
- Certain yoga moves also strengthen these muscles, so if you are struggling with doing this regularly or have considered taking up yoga for a while, this may be a good time to start.
- Imagine your lungs are in the pelvis and relax perineum on inhale and draw up on exhale.

Warnings:

- Always do kegels with an empty bladder. Doing kegels during urination can weaken your pelvic floor and increase your risk of contracting a urinary tract infection.

- Don't do kegels while urinating, except to locate the muscles initially. Interrupting urine flow can result in kidney and bladder problems.

SWIMMING

Swimming is a low-impact, full-body workout that can help improve cardiovascular health, endurance, and muscle tone. It can also be an enjoyable and stress-reducing activity, which may positively influence sexual desire and performance.

Swimming is not only beneficial for your physical health and well-being but it can improve your sex life. Swimming can boost your libido and sexual performance in addition to toning your body, improving your cardiac function and increasing your energy levels. It is a great way to get back into exercising following surgery, injury, heart attack or if you have a disability which impacts upon your movement and ability to exercise, as the water supports the body.

Swimming in a horizontal position places less exertion on your body because the heart isn't working against gravity: therefore, it doesn't have to work as hard to pump blood around your body, according to Professor Brent Rusthall, Professor of Exercise and Nutritional Sciences at San Diego University.

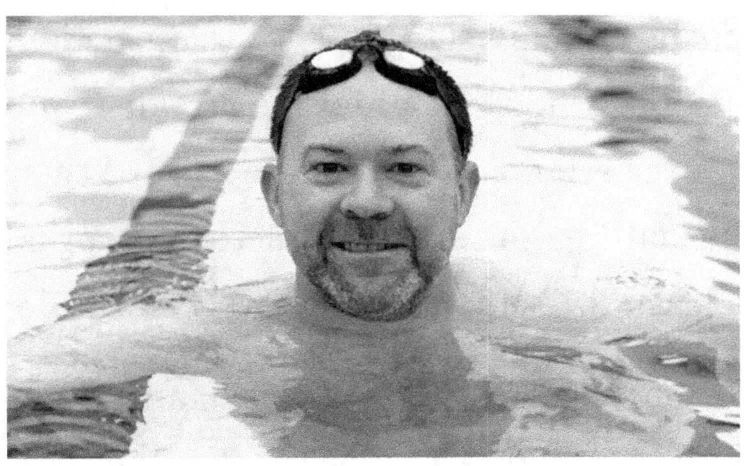

A Harvard University study of 160 male and female swimmers in their 40s and 60s found a positive relationship between physical exercise and sexual intercourse. The swimmers in their 60s reported having sex lives similar to that of people aged 40+ in the general population (Krucoff and Krucoff 2000). Bortz and Wallace (1999) found that the fitter an older person was, the better their sexual activity and satisfaction. People who look after their bodies and exercise tend to be more aware of their sexual health, enjoying increased sexual pleasure.

According to swimming coach and pilates expert Agneta Lindberg, it's the best exercise to tone your pelvic floor muscles leading to more powerful orgasms and heightening the sexual experience of your partner. Strengthening your pelvic floor muscles can also help alleviate health problems such as urinary incontinence and vaginal prolapse.

What strokes are best?

The best stroke for your pelvic floor is the breast stroke as the simple action of bringing your legs together causes your thigh and pelvic floor muscles to contract, thus strengthening them. All swimming strokes help to tone your waist and pelvic muscles to some degree because you constantly have to engage these muscles in order to keep your balance as you swim.

Studies have found that the heart rate of a swimmer is 12 beats per minute less on average than that of a runner, enabling you to keep up intensity for longer, thus increasing the benefits of your workout. This in turn improves stamina and energy levels, both of which are beneficial to enjoying sexual intercourse.

The temperature of the water prevents you from becoming as overheated as someone working out on land, which enables you to work out at the same intensity for a longer period of time, thus building stamina.

Long term benefits

Like all exercise, swimming boosts your endorphins, feel good hormones, which can help to increase your libido by reducing your stress levels – a major contributory factor in low libido.

Swimming can improve brain function through a process known as hippocampal neurogenesis, whereby the brain replaces cells destroyed as a result of the effects of stress upon the body.

It can also improve your circulation, increasing blood flow around the body and especially to the genital area, boosting sexual function.

Exercising in general has psychological benefits to health by reducing stress, raising self-esteem, improving your mood and increasing self-confidence, all of which can contribute to a more enriched sex life.

Having a swimmer's body is also seen as a desirable image. When researchers at Cambridge University showed 700 women 30 different male body types, they found that the most attractive image was that of a swimmer: broad shoulders, nipped-in waist and small hips. Having a swimmer's physique is also beneficial for women: you can balance out a pear-shaped figure by developing your upper body using breaststroke to tone chest muscles, which increases support to the breasts making them look firmer and uplifted, and tone thighs, making them look thinner.

Swimming is a low impact activity putting less strain on joints and limbs and keeps you looking young. Jogging has been found to increase the risk of wrinkles as the upwards and downwards motion of running causes the elastic fibres in our face to stretch. People who run or jog often have a gaunt, thin face that can look older. Swimmers do not burn as much fat as runners but generally develop an all over body muscle tone, rather than just their legs. This is why swimmers tend to have bodies which look more balanced and in proportion because of the large number of muscles they use and the range of movements involved in swimming strokes.

Summer is an excellent time to go swimming, especially in outside pools and the sea, so take advantage of the warm weather and feel the benefits that swimming can have on your sexual pleasure. If you continue to swim long after you have returned from your summer holiday, you can boost your sex life all year long.

YOGA EXERCISES

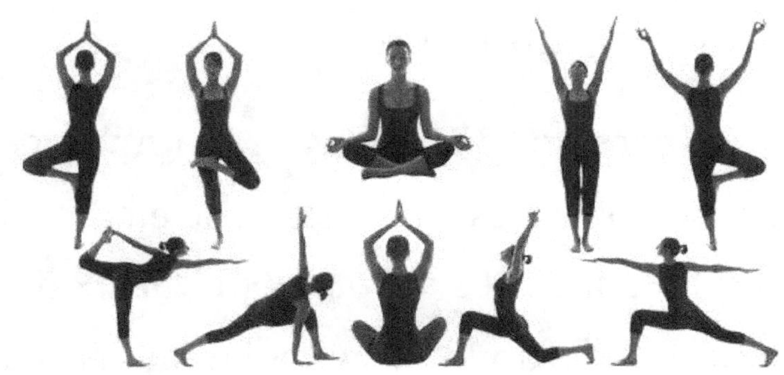

Yoga, an ancient practice that originated in India, is known for its numerous physical, mental, and spiritual benefits. When it comes to improving sex performance, yoga can be a powerful tool. By promoting physical fitness, relaxation, mindfulness, and stress reduction, yoga can positively impact various aspects of sexual health and enhance overall sexual experience. Let's explore in detail how yoga exercises can boost sex performance:

1.   Increased Flexibility: Yoga involves a series of poses that gently stretch and lengthen muscles throughout the body. Improved flexibility can lead to increased range of motion during sex, making it easier to engage in different positions and movements comfortably.

2.   Enhanced Circulation: Yoga poses often focus on opening up the chest, hips, and pelvis. These movements help to improve blood circulation throughout the body, including the genital area. Better blood flow can lead to stronger and more

sustained erections in men and increased sensitivity in women.

3.   Strengthening Core and Pelvic Floor Muscles: Many yoga poses require engaging the core and pelvic floor muscles to maintain balance and stability. Strengthening these muscles can lead to better control over sexual functions, such as maintaining erections and delaying ejaculation in men and increasing vaginal tone and control in women.

4.   Stress Reduction: Chronic stress and anxiety can negatively impact sexual desire and performance. Yoga incorporates mindfulness and deep breathing techniques that activate the

body's relaxation response, reducing stress hormones like cortisol and promoting a sense of calm. Lower stress levels can lead to increased libido and better sexual functioning.

5. Mind-Body Connection: Yoga encourages practitioners to be fully present in the moment and to connect with their bodies and sensations. Developing a stronger mind-body connection can improve body awareness during sex, allowing individuals to better understand their desires and respond to their partner's cues.

6. Improved Endurance and Stamina: Yoga is a form of exercise that builds strength and endurance over time. As

practitioners progress in their practice, they may notice increased stamina during physical activities, including sexual intercourse.

7.   Balancing Hormones: Certain yoga poses, particularly inversions, are believed to help balance hormonal levels in the body. Hormonal imbalances can contribute to sexual issues, such as low libido and erectile dysfunction, and yoga may aid in restoring hormonal equilibrium.

8.   Boosting Confidence and Body Image: Regular yoga practice can help improve body confidence and self-esteem. Feeling more comfortable in one's body can lead to greater sexual

confidence and a willingness to explore new experiences with a partner.

9. Emotional Well-being: Yoga is known to have a positive impact on mental health, reducing symptoms of anxiety and depression. Better emotional well-being can lead to a more satisfying and enjoyable sexual experience.

The most common types of yoga

1. Vinyasa yoga

Vinyasa means "to place in a special way" and, in this case, yoga postures. Vinyasa yoga is often considered the most athletic yoga style, and was adapted from ashtanga yoga in the 1980s. Many types of yoga can also be considered "vinyasa flows," such as ashtanga, power yoga, and prana.

In vinyasa classes, movements are coordinated with your breath in order to flow from one pose to another. Vinyasa styles can vary depending on the teacher, and there can be many types of poses in different sequences. I personally teach an alignment-based style of vinyasa and choreograph new flows every time, but I also like to hold some of the poses a bit longer after warming up.

VINYASA YOGA POSES

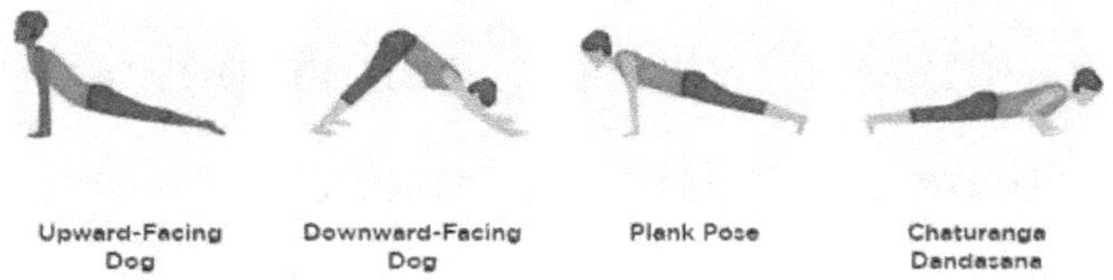

2. Hatha yoga

The Sanskrit term "hatha" is an umbrella term for all physical postures of yoga. In the West, hatha yoga simply refers to all the other styles of yoga (ashtanga, Iyengar, etc.) that are grounded in a physical practice. However, there are other branches of yoga such as kriya, raja, and karma yoga that are separate from the physical-based yoga practice.

The physical-based yoga is the most popular and has numerous styles.

Hatha yoga classes are best for beginners since they are usually paced slower than other yoga styles. Hatha classes today are a classic approach to breathing and exercises. If you are brand-new to yoga, hatha yoga is a great entry point to the practice.

3. Iyengar yoga

Iyengar yoga was founded by B.K.S. Iyengar focuses on alignment as well as detailed and precise movements. In an Iyengar class, students perform a variety of postures while controlling the breath.

Generally, poses are held for a long time while adjusting the minutiae of the pose. Iyengar relies heavily on props to help students perfect their form and go deeper into poses in a safe manner. Although you won't jump around, you will definitely get a workout and feel incredibly open and relaxed after an Iyengar class. This style is really great for people with injuries who need to work slowly and methodically.

4. Kundalini yoga

Kundalini yoga practice is equal parts spiritual and physical. This style is all about releasing the kundalini energy in your body said to be trapped, or coiled, in the lower spine.

A kundalini class will really work your core and breath with fast-moving, invigorating postures and breath exercises. These classes are pretty intense and can involve chanting, mantra, and meditation. To learn more about this specific practice, check out our kundalini yoga explainer.

5. Ashtanga yoga

In Sanskrit, ashtanga is translated as "Eight Limb path." In Mysore, India, people gather to practice this form of yoga together at their own pace—if you see Mysore-led ashtanga, it's expected of you to know the series. Vinyasa yoga stems from ashtanga as the flowing style linking breath to movement. To learn more about this specific practice, check out our beginner's guide to ashtanga yoga.

Ashtanga yoga involves a very physically demanding sequence of postures, so this style of yoga is definitely not for the beginner. It takes an experienced yogi to really love it. Ashtanga starts with five sun salutation A's and five sun salutation B's and then moves into a series of standing and floor postures.

6. Bikram yoga

Bikram yoga is named after Bikram Choudhury and features a sequence of set poses in a sauna-like room—typically set to 105 degrees and 40% humidity. Choudhury faced sexual assault and harassment lawsuits in the U.S. and fled to Mexico in 2017. Many studios that were formerly Bikram now practice hot yoga, in an effort to disassociate with the founder.

The sequence never changes and includes a series of 26 basic postures, with each one performed twice. Many of these poses are focused on proper alignment. If you're interested in yoga with the heat turned up, look for studios that offer hot yoga classes.

7. Yin yoga

Yin yoga is a slow-paced style of yoga with seated postures that are held for longer periods of time. Yin can also be a meditative yoga practice that helps you find inner peace.

Yin is a great class for beginners, as postures can be held anywhere from 45 seconds to 2 minutes. The classes are relaxed, as you're supposed to let gravity do most of the work.

8. Restorative yoga

Restorative yoga focuses on winding down after a long day and relaxing your mind. At its core, this style focuses on body relaxation. Restorative yoga also helps to cleanse and free your mind.

You'll spend more time in fewer postures throughout a restorative yoga class. Many of the poses are modified to be easier and more relaxing. Like Iyengar, many props are used and placed just right, such as blankets, bolsters, and eye pillows. All of the props are there to help you sink deeper into relaxation.

9. Prenatal yoga

Prenatal yoga is carefully adapted for moms-to-be, and is tailored to women in all trimesters. Many have said that prenatal is one of the best types of exercise for expectant moms because of the pelvic floor work, focus on breathing, and bonding with the growing baby. Prenatal yoga also helps mothers prepare for labor and delivery.

During this practice, you'll use props in order to modify your poses and ensure stability—in this class, its way more about stability than flexibility.

10. Anusara yoga

Anusara is a modern-day version of hatha yoga, most similar to vinyasa in that it focuses on alignment, but with more emphasis on the mind-body-heart connection. It was founded by John Friend who created a unique system called the Universal Principles of

Alignment. He resigned in 2012 after accusations of sexual misconduct and financial mismanagement. Friend has since partnered with Desi and Micah Springer to teach the Bowspring method.

Anusara focuses on spirals and how each body part should be moving, and it's also known for its emphasis on heart opening. Expect to stop in class and gather around a student as the instructor breaks down a pose.

11. Jivamukti yoga

Jivamukti was founded in 1984 by Sharon Ganon and David Life. Jivamukti is mainly vinyasa-flow-style classes infused with Hindu spiritual teachings.

At its core, this style emphasizes connection to Earth as a living being, so most Jivamukti devotees follow a vegetarian philosophy.

It is essential to remember that yoga is not a quick fix for sexual performance issues, and individual results may vary. Consistent and dedicated practice over time, combined with a holistic approach to overall health and lifestyle, can lead to the best results. Additionally, yoga can complement other forms of physical activity and healthy habits, such as a balanced diet and regular exercise, to support sexual health and overall well-being. As with any exercise program, it's essential to listen to your body, practice safely, and consult with a healthcare professional if you have any specific health concerns or medical conditions.

CONCLUSION

Remember that maintaining a healthy lifestyle goes beyond just exercise. A balanced diet, adequate sleep, stress management, and avoiding harmful habits like smoking and excessive alcohol consumption are also important factors that can support men's sexual health.

As with any exercise program, it's essential to consult with a healthcare professional before starting a new regimen, especially if you have any pre-existing medical conditions. They can provide personalized advice and ensure that the chosen exercises are safe and suitable for your individual needs.